Brown

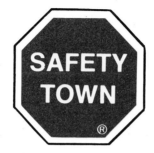

Poisons
Make You Sick

By Dorothy Chlad

Illustrated by Lydia Halverson

 CHILDRENS PRESS ®
CHICAGO

Library of Congress Cataloging in Publication Data

Chlad, Dorothy.
   Poisons make you sick.

   (Safety Town)
   Summary: A small girl named Tammy explains why one
should never put strange things in one's mouth.
   1. Poisons—Juvenile literature.   2.   Toxicology—
Juvenile literature. [1. Poisons 2. Health. 3. Safety.]
I. Halverson, Lydia, ill.   II. Title.   III. Series:
Chlad, Dorothy.   Safety Town.
RA1214.C45   1984   615.9'05   83-24029
ISBN O-516-O1976-7   AACR2

Hi, my name is
Tammy.

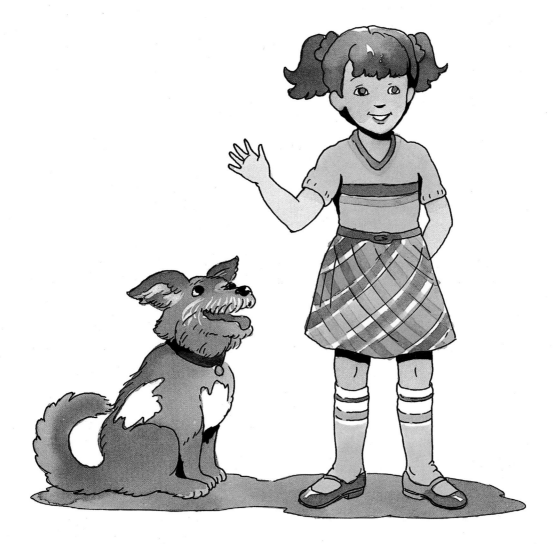

I want to tell you
about poisons.

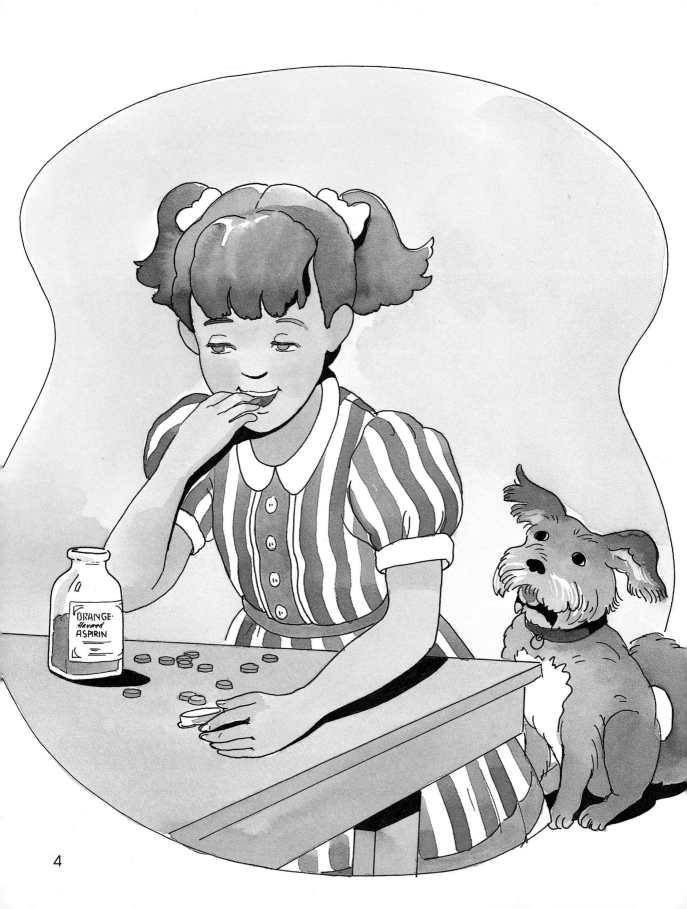

One day I ate a lot
of pills. I thought they
were orange candies.

They made me very
sick. They had poison
in them.

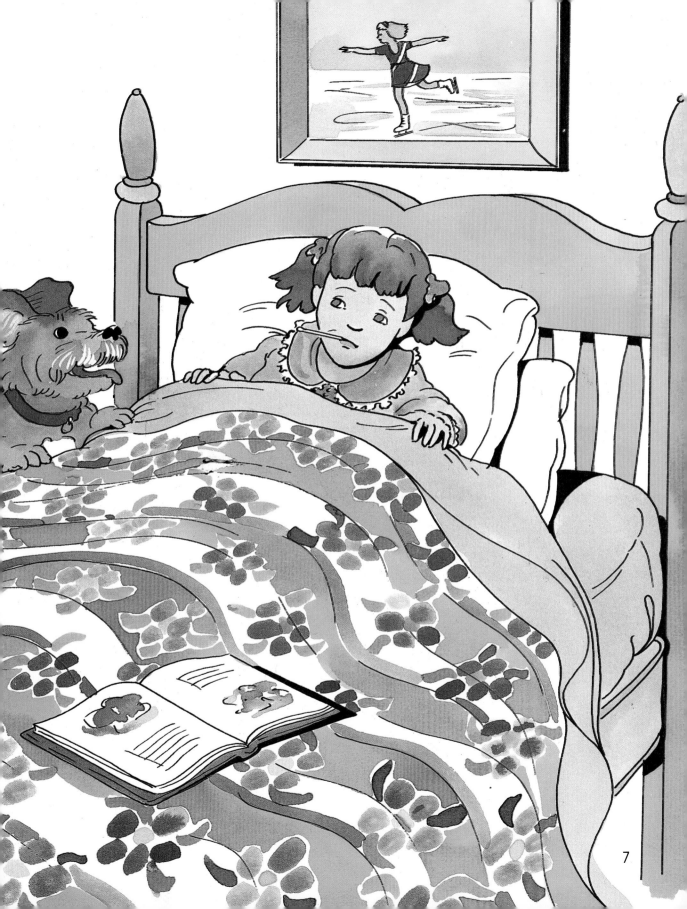

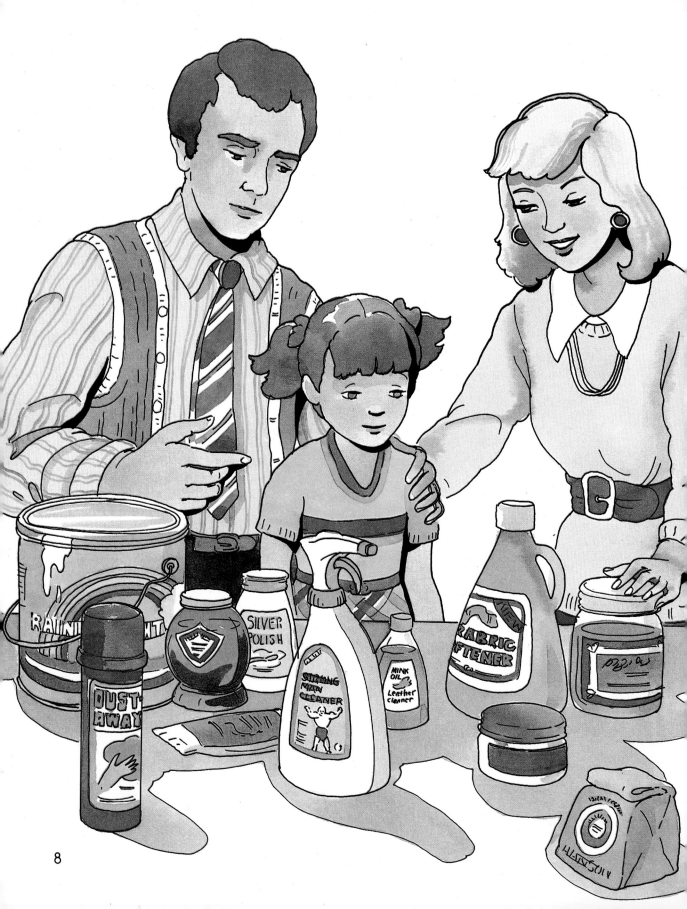

Now. . . I never put
strange things in my
mouth until I ask
mom and dad about
them.

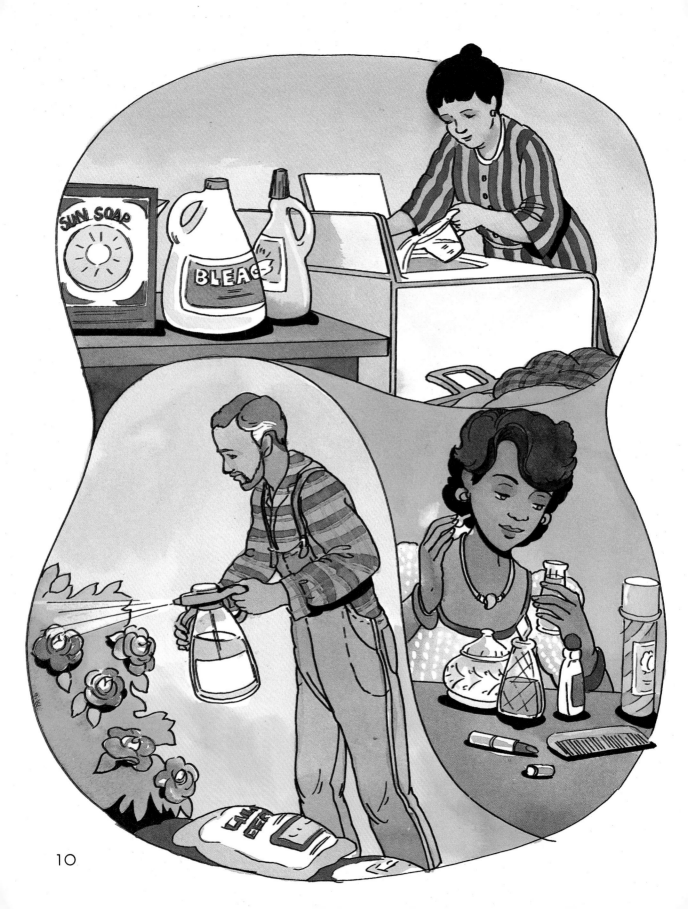

Many things have
poison in them.

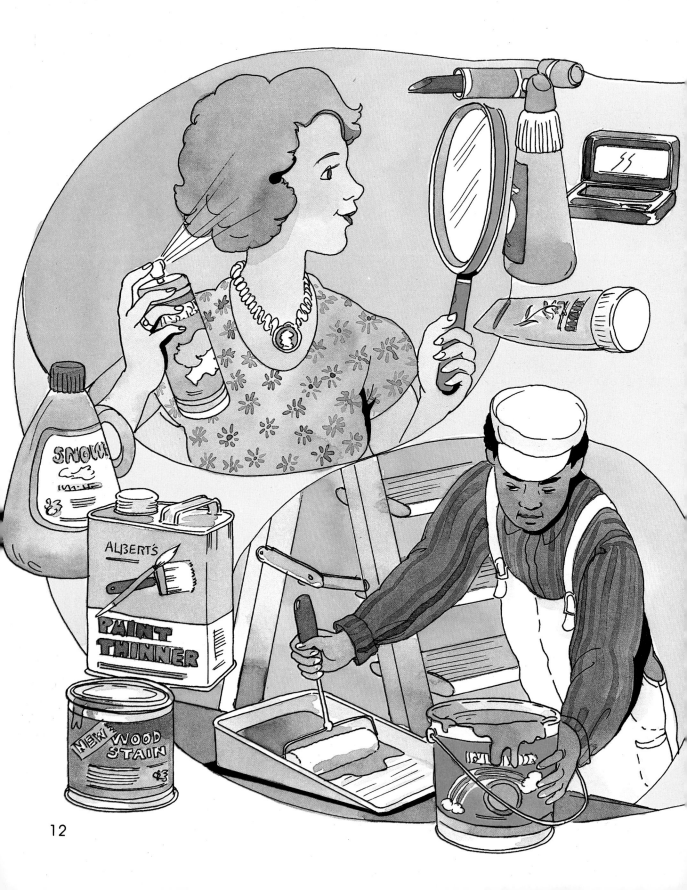

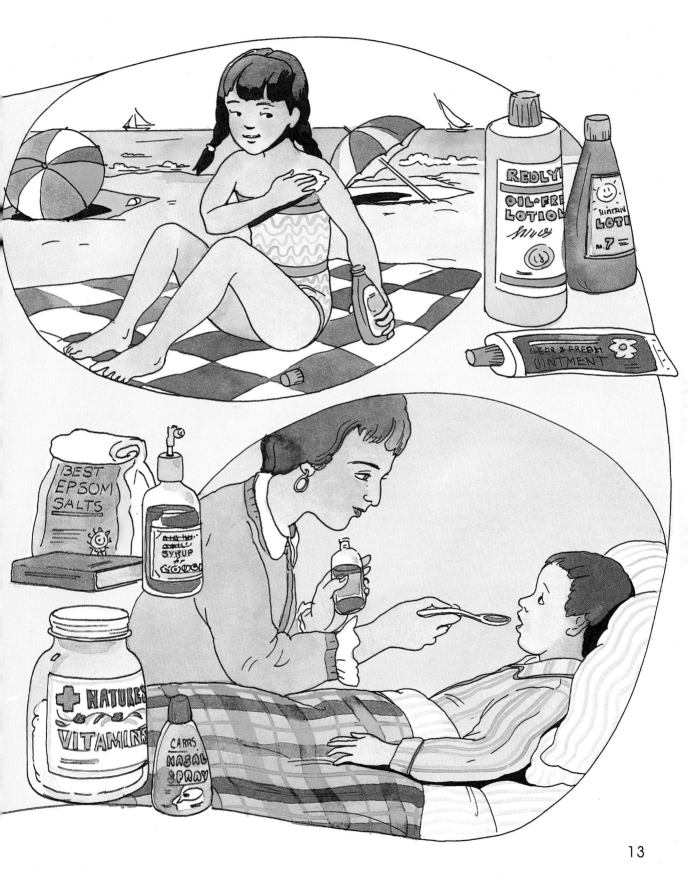

Even things that smell and taste good, may have poison in them.

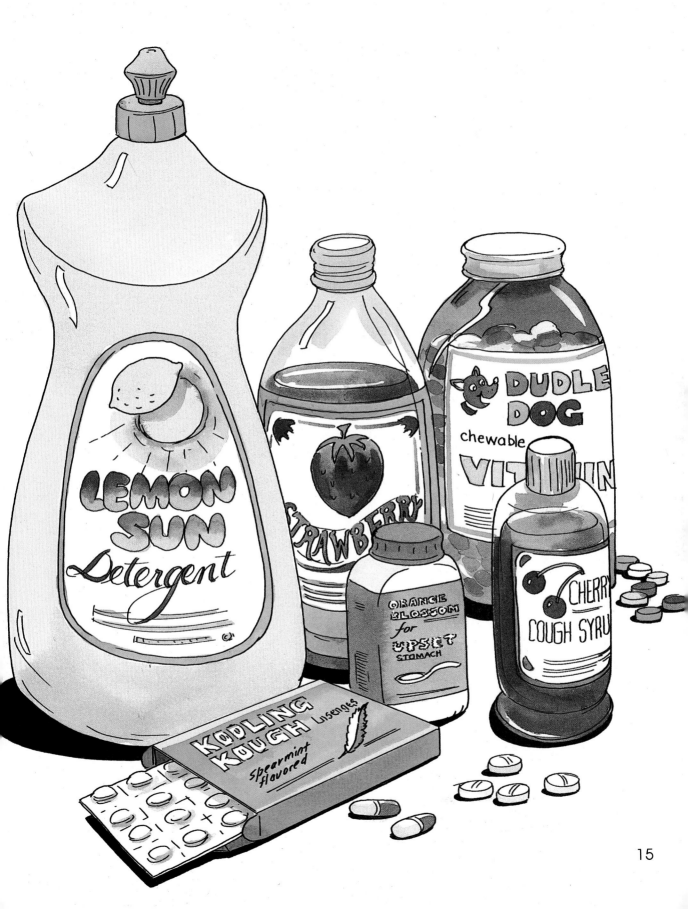

15

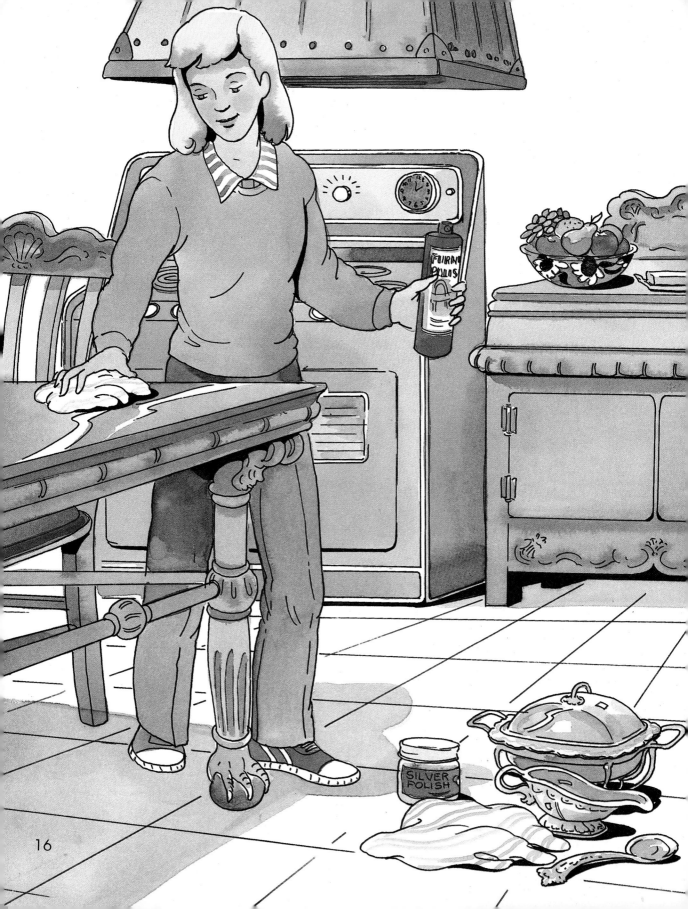

My mom and dad
need some of these to
keep our house clean.

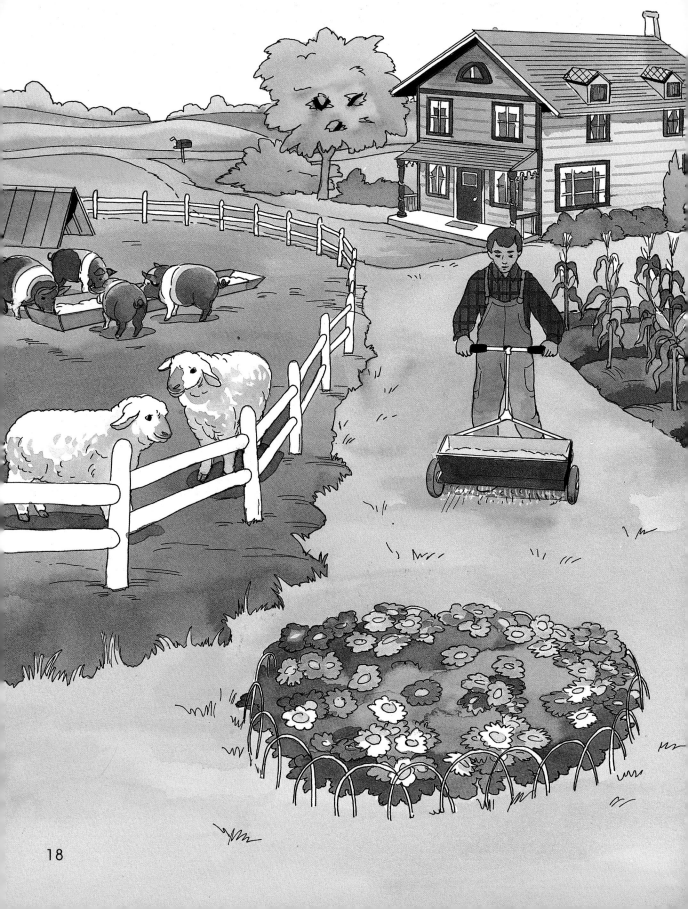

Our friends need
some of these things to
help food, flowers, and
animals grow.

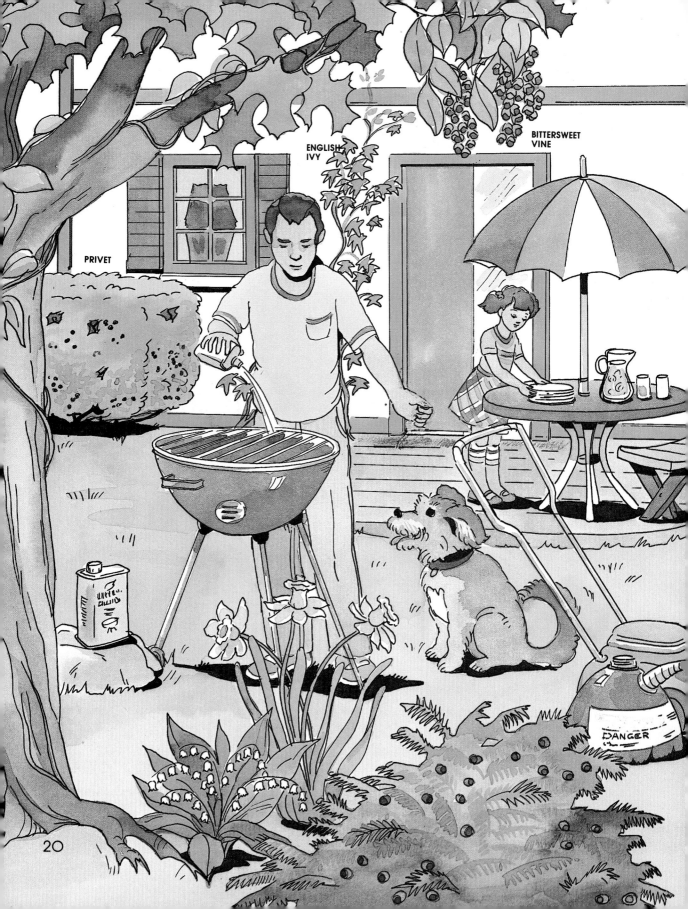

ENGLISH
IVY

BITTERSWEET
VINE

PRIVET

DANGER

20

Many things that grow outdoors have poison in them.

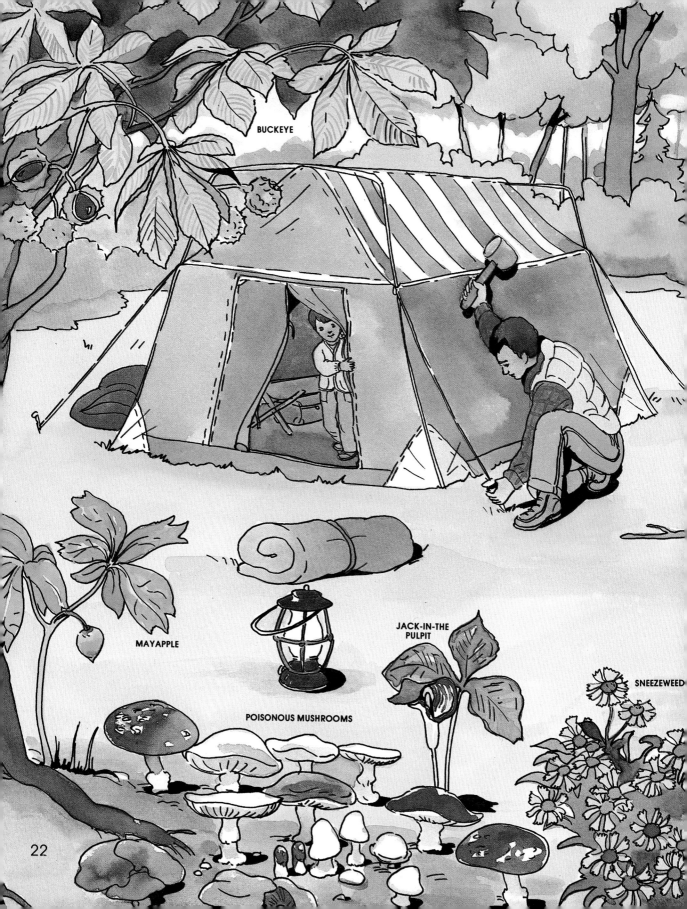

BUCKEYE

MAYAPPLE

JACK-IN-THE-PULPIT

SNEEZEWEED

POISONOUS MUSHROOMS

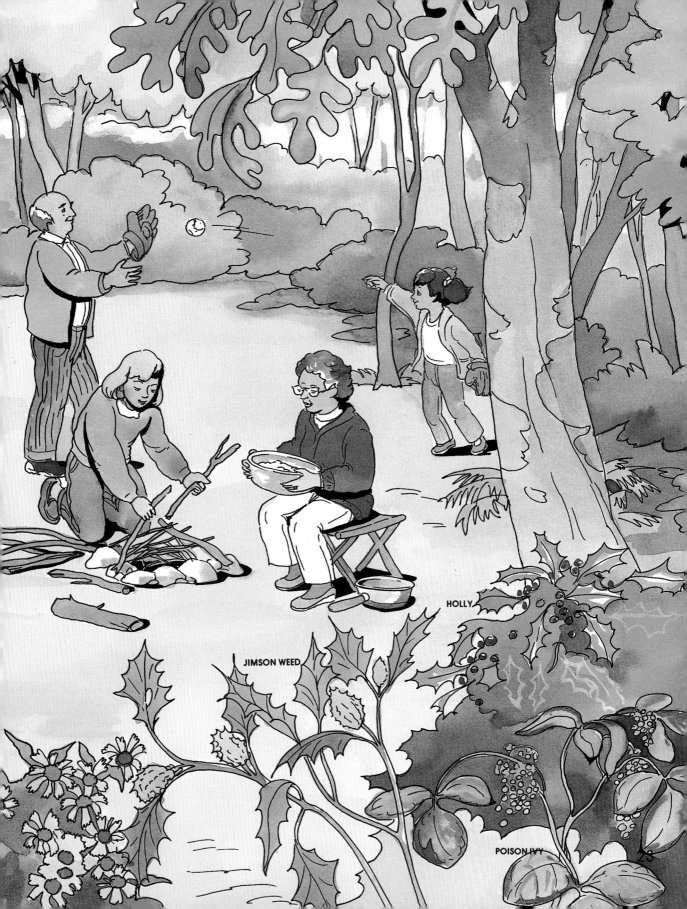

HOLLY

JIMSON WEED

POISON IVY

25

Be careful. Wherever you are. . . in the house . . . in the garage. . . or outdoors

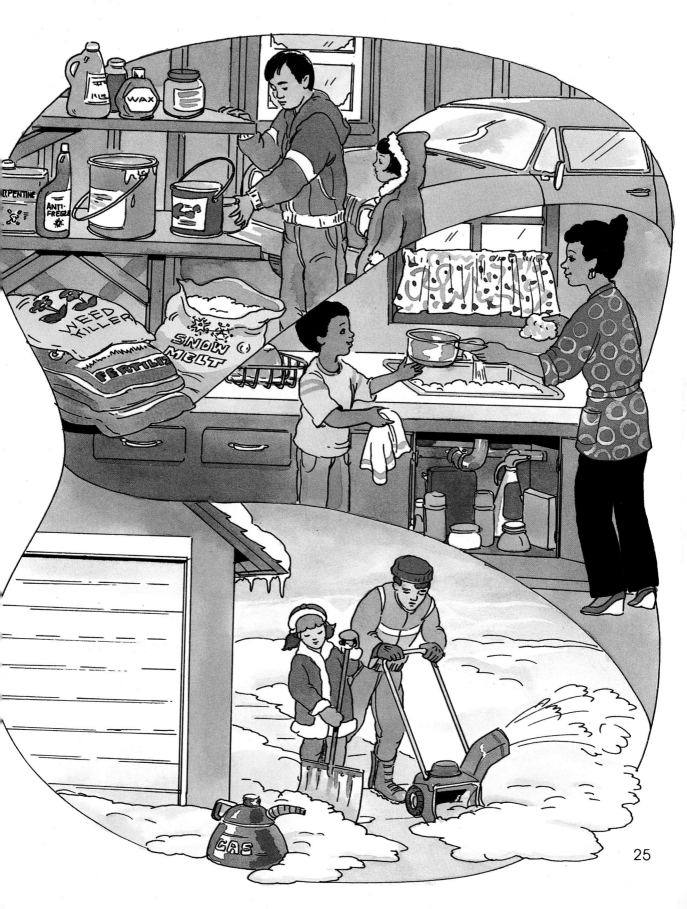

25

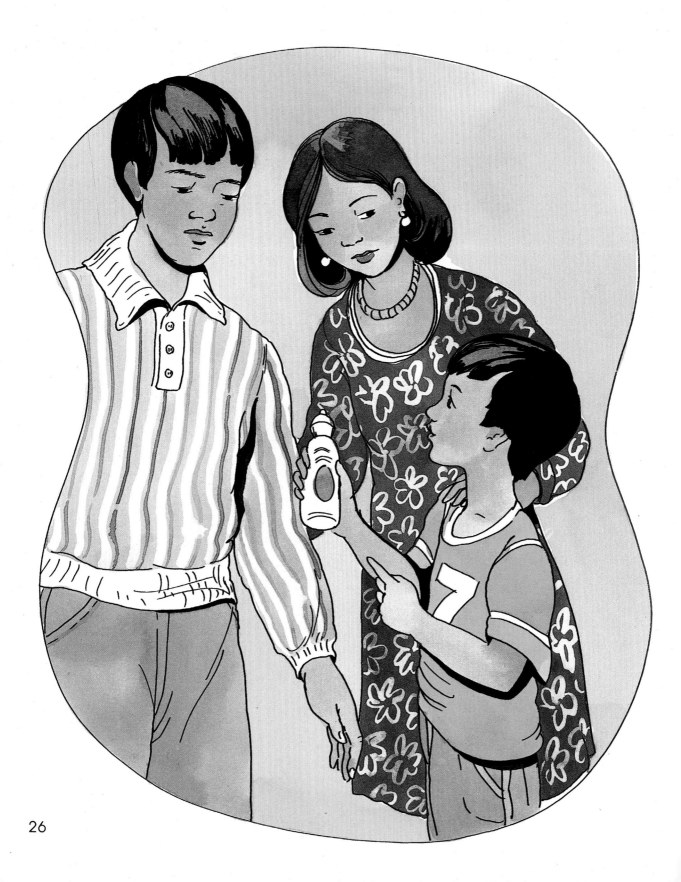

. . . always ask mom or dad before putting anything strange in your mouth.

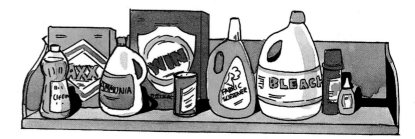

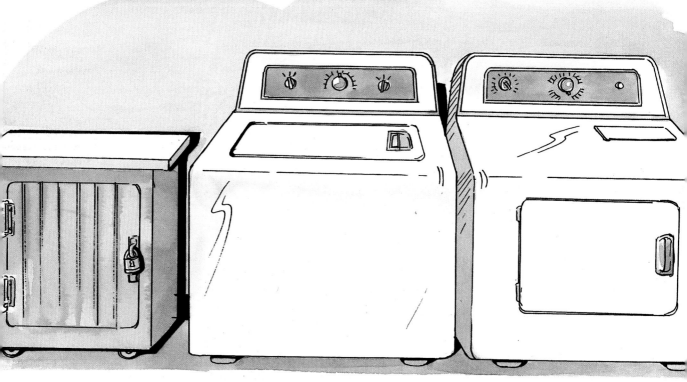

Watch out for things
that are poison.
Ask your mom or
dad to put poison

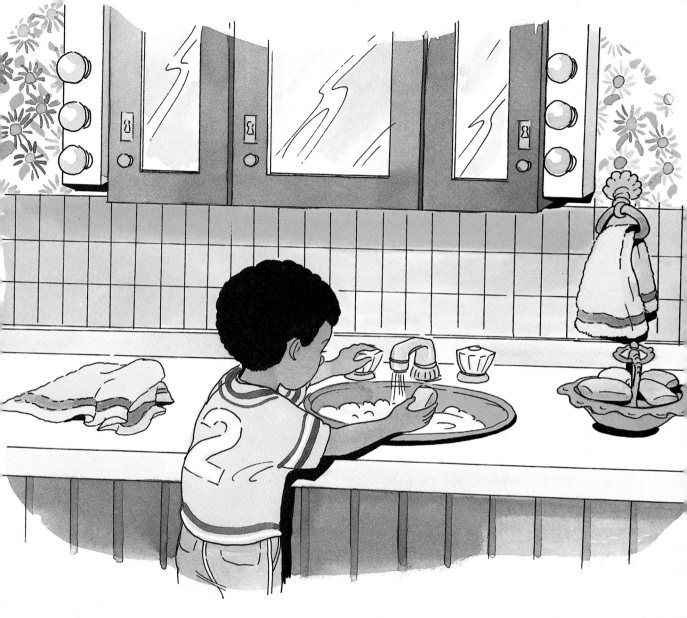

things on a high shelf
or in a locked cabinet.
Then your younger
sister or brother cannot
get to them.

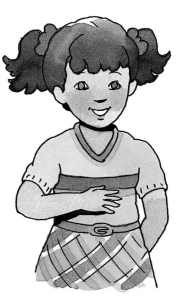

If you remember these rules, you will not get sick.

1. Many things have poison in them.

2. Some things that smell and taste good have poison in them.

3. Always ask mom or dad questions before you put anything strange in your mouth.

4. Ask your mom and dad to put poison things on a high shelf or in a locked cabinet.

About the Author

Dorothy Chlad, founder of the total concept of Safety Town, is recognized internationally as a leader in Preschool/Early Childhood Safety Education. She has authored eight books on the program, and has conducted the only workshops dedicated to the concept. Under Mrs. Chlad's direction, the National Safety Town Center was founded to promote the program through community involvement.

She has presented the importance of safety education at local, state, and national safety and education conferences, such as National Community Education Association, National Safety Council, and the American Driver and Traffic Safety Education Association. She serves as a member of several national committees, such as the Highway Traffic Safety Division and the Educational Resources Division of National Safety Council. Chlad was an active participant at the Sixth International Conference on Safety Education.

Dorothy Chlad continues to serve as a consultant for State Departments of Safety and Education. She has also consulted for the TV program, "Sesame Street" and recently wrote this series of safety books for Childrens Press.

A participant of White House Conferences on safety, Dorothy Chlad has received numerous honors and awards including National Volunteer Activist and YMCA Career Woman of Achievement. In 1983, Dorothy Chlad was one of sixty people nationally to receive the **President's Volunteer Action Award** from President Reagan for twenty years of Safety Town efforts.

About the Artist

Lydia Halverson was born Lydia Geretti in midtown Manhattan. When she was two, her parents left New York and moved to Italy. Four years later her family returned to the United States and settled in the Chicago Area. Lydia attended the University of Illinois, graduating with a degree in fine arts. She worked as a graphic designer for many years before finally concentrating on book illustration.

Lydia lives with her husband and two cats in a suburb of Chicago and is active in several environmental organizations.